"Kali - finger interlaced Mudra" indeed (handwritten)

Mud[ras]

finding a fo. *[pure] energy & overcoming difficulty* (handwritten)

Awakening Chakras

19 Simple Hand Gestures for Awakening & Balancing your Chakras

by

Advait

Disclaimer and FTC Notice

Mudras for Awakening Chakras: 19 Simple Hand Gestures for Awakening and Balancing Your Chakras
Copyright © 2014, Advait. All rights reserved.

ISBN-13: 978-1511896641

ISBN-10:1511896647

Advait

Free 7 Day email course

"Sukshma Asanas for Awakening Chakras"

The Mudras in themselves are a very effective technique for Chakra Awakening. But, do you know that you can increase the effectiveness of these Mudras, manifolds?

Let me explain how...

Yogic philosophy puts a lot of emphasis on the concept of Action (karm) and Inaction (akarm).

These concepts have great philosophical as well as physical implications.

On a physical level, according to yoga, action followed by inaction gives greater and far more effective results.

'Action' acts as a *stimulant* and then 'Inaction' acts as a *re-enforcement*.

In this case,

Mudras represent inaction, and when you perform certain micro-exercises called as "Sukshma Asanas", which represent action, before practicing the Mudras, the effect and intensity of Mudras increase exponentially.

In simple terms; performing sukshma asanas before practicing the Mudras works wonders.

I have compiled 7 such sukshma asanas, one for each chakra, into a 7 day email course.

And, I am offering the online email course, for **FREE** to my readers only.

Get your Free 7 day email course; **"Sukshma Asanas for Awakening Chakras"** here:

https://goo.gl/nRWLb

Simply type the link in your web browser to get the free email course and fast track your Chakra Awakening process.

-Advait

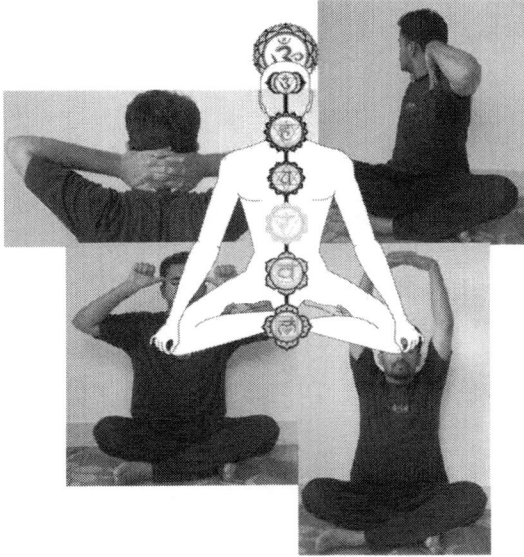

Mudras for Awakening Chakras

Contents

What are Mudras?

According to the Vedic culture of ancient India, our entire world is made of 'the five elements' called as *The Panch-Maha-Bhuta's*. The five elements being **Earth**, **Water**, **Fire**, **Wind** and **Space/Vacuum**. They are also called the earth element, water element, fire element, wind element and space element.

These five elements constitute the human body – the nutrients from the soil (earth) are absorbed by the plants which we consume (thus we survive on the earth element), the blood flowing through own veins represents the water element, the body heat represents the fire element, the oxygen we inhale and the carbon dioxide we exhale represents the wind element and the sinuses we have in our nose and skull represent the space element.

As long as these five elements in our body are balanced and maintain appropriate levels we remain healthy. An imbalance of these elements in the human body leads to a deteriorated health and diseases.

Now understand this, the command and control center of all these five elements lies in our fingers. So literally, our health lies at our fingertips.

The Mudra healing method that I am going to teach you depends on our fingers.

To understand this, we should first know the finger-element relationship:

Thumb – Fire element.

Index finger – Wind element.

Middle finger – Space/Vacuum element.

Third finger – Earth element.

Small finger – Water element.

This image will give you a better understanding of the concept:

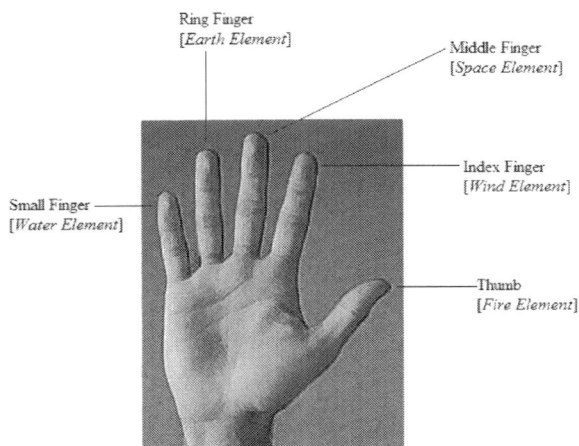

Ring Finger
[*Earth Element*]

Middle Finger
[*Space Element*]

Index Finger
[*Wind Element*]

Small Finger
[*Water Element*]

Thumb
[*Fire Element*]

When the fingers are brought together in a specific pattern and are touched to each other, or slightly pressed against each other, the formation is called as a '*Mudra*'.

When the five fingers are touched and pressed in a peculiar way to form a Mudra, it affects the levels of the five elements in our body, thus balancing those elements and inducing good health.

P.S. The Mudra Healing Methods aren't just theory or wordplay; these are healing methods from the ancient Indian Vedic culture, proven and tested over ages.

Mudras for Awakening Chakras

Important

Read this before you read any further

For the better understanding of the reader, detail images have been provided for every mudra along with the method to perform it.

Most of the Mudras given in this book are to be performed using both your hands, but the Mudras whose images show only one hand performing the Mudra, are to be performed simultaneously on both your hands for the Mudras to have the maximum effect.

What are Chakras?

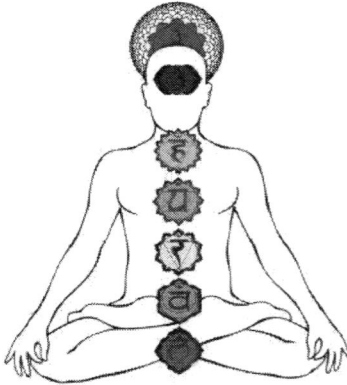

7. The Crown Chakra

6. The Third Eye Chakra

5. The Throat Chakra

4. The Heart Chakra

3. The Solar Plexus Chakra

2. The Sacral Chakra

1. The Base/Root Chakra

I want to keep this book absolutely fluff free, so, I will not talk about how Chakras are the metaphysical entities that are essential for spiritual awakening and how they take you closer to The Divine One and keep you at peace. All I want to do is to make you understand that by awakening and balancing your Chakras you will achieve everlasting health, physically and emotionally and that this book is the best Medical Insurance you ever bought!

"Energy can neither be created nor can it be destroyed, it only changes from one form to another."

The Human body needs energy to sustain life, this essential energy is obtained in two ways:

The Physical mode – The food we consume and the air we breathe cause a physical combustion of food and the assimilation of essential nutrients which provide us with the energy we need for survival.

The Meta-physical mode – The Omnipresent Universal Life energy is absorbed or channeled into our body.

This Universal Life energy enters the human body at Seven specific points, located on the spine, these points are THE CHAKRAS.

Simply put, The Seven Chakras are the inlet energy taps of the human body.

All these Chakras are associated with certain Glands and Vital Organs and the energy entering the Chakras is lead to them for proper functioning and nourishment.

If a Chakra is Closed, Blocked or Un-Balanced then these Vital Organs and Glands are malnourished leading to further complications and diseases. (Both on a physical and meta-physical level)

For example: If The Anaahat Chakra (The Heart Chakra) is blocked or unbalanced then the person is prone to cardiovascular disorders and also to emotional instability.

A person whose Chakras are awakened and in a balanced state will be in the best of his health. Also, a consistent harmony between the Chakras will induce a feeling of prosperity, well being and satisfaction. Such a person can only look forward to spiritual awakening and eternal bliss.

Now, let's get down to business, and awaken & balance your Chakras.

Muladhaar Chakra / The Root Chakra

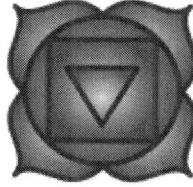

Sanskrit Name:

मूलाधार चक्र - Muladhaar chakra

English Name:

The Root Chakra

Symbol:
Lotus with four petals.

Colour:
Red.

Location:

It is Located at the base of the spine.

Element:
Earth element.

Glands it Controls:
Gonads and Adrenal Medulla.

Organs it Controls:
Rectum, Kidneys, and Organs in lower abdomen.

Food that nourishes this Chakra:
Red Meat, Spinach, Spices and Pepper.

The Root Chakra is located at the base of the spine, hence the name. It is associated and responsible for the health of the digestive track, intestines and the lower abdominal organs. When this Chakra is balanced, you will feel at peace, confident and secure.

Mudras for Awakening & Balancing Muladhaar Chakra / The Root Chakra

While performing these Mudras, Concentrate on your breathing and visualize a ray of bright Red light entering your Root Chakra and the Chakra glowing in a bright Red Luminescence.

MuladhaarChakramudra / Mudra of Root Chakra

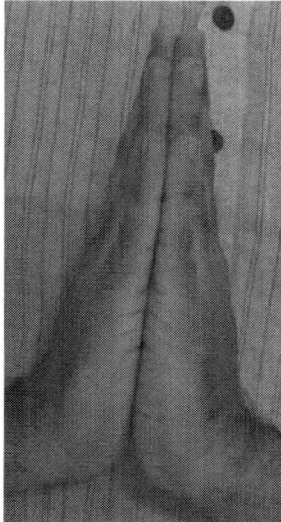

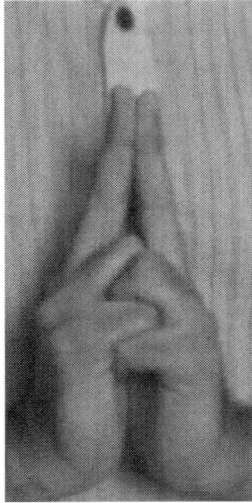

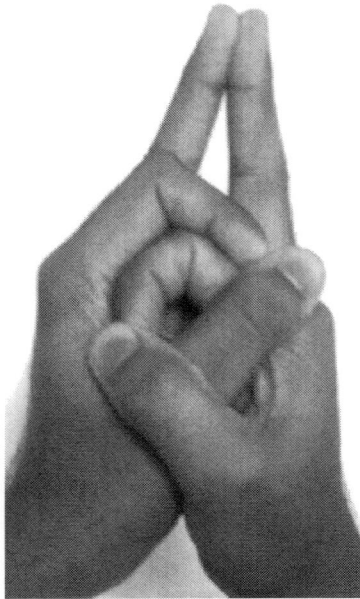

Mudras for Awakening Chakras

Method:

This Mudra has to be performed in a seating position.

Be seated comfortably in an upright posture and concentrate on your breathing to relax.

Join both the palms together like in the Indian salutation 'Namaste'.

Then interlace and bend the Ring fingers and the Little fingers of both the hands (see to it that the fingers are folded inwards, within the palms).

Extend out the Middle fingers and join the tips of both the Middle fingers and press slightly.

Now join the tips of the Index fingers to the tips of the Thumbs, forming interlocking circles (Refer the image).

This Mudra is to be held in front of your pubic bone.

While you are doing this Mudra, simultaneously keep contracting your Perineal floor muscle (Refer the image).

(Don't keep the muscle contracted but keep clenching and relaxing this muscle continuously)

Duration:

This Mudra should be performed till you feel tired by clenching and relaxing your Perineal muscle. Take rest then repeat a couple of times.

This Mudra should be performed twice a day, once in the morning and once in the evening for best results.

Mushtimudra / Mudra of Fist

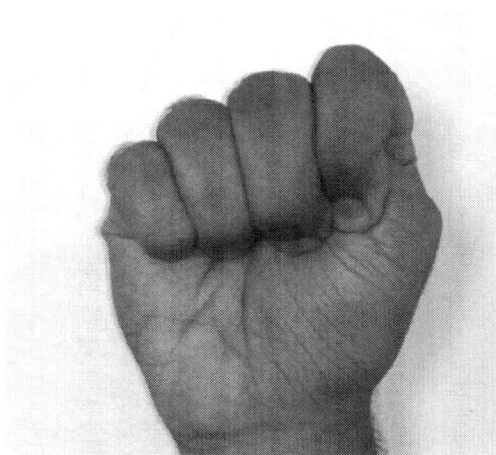

Method:

This Mudra has to be performed in a seating position.

Be seated comfortably in an upright posture and concentrate on your breathing to relax.

Touch the tip of your thumb to the base of the Ring finger and press slightly.

Close all the other fingers over the Thumb to form a fist.

(Refer the image)

Form this Mudra on each hand and rest the fists against the lower belly.

Duration:

This Mudra should be performed for at least 5 minutes and can be performed for 40 minutes at a stretch.

This Mudra should be performed twice a day, once in the morning and once in the evening for best results.

Gadamudra / Mudra of Spear

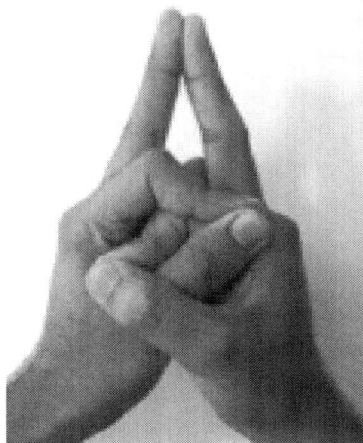

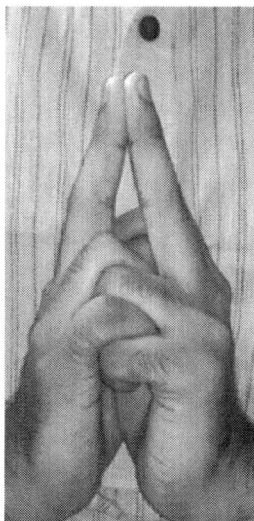

Method:

This Mudra has to be performed in a seating position.

Be seated comfortably in an upright posture and concentrate on your breathing to relax.

Form two interlacing rings by touching the tips of your index fingers with the tips of your thumbs as shown in the image.

Keep the Middle fingers straight and pointing upwards, and then touch the upright middle fingers to each other.

The final step is to interlace the ring fingers and the little fingers together, and bend them in the second knuckle such that there tips point downwards.

This Mudra should be held in front of your lower abdomen and not at chest height.

Duration:

This Mudra should be performed for at least 5 minutes and can be performed for 40 minutes at a stretch.

This Mudra should be performed twice a day, once in the morning and once in the evening for best results.

Svadhishtaana Chakra / The Sacral Chakra

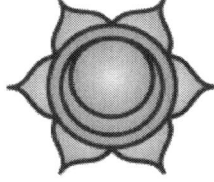

Sanskrit Name:

स्वाधष्ठिान चक्र - Svadhistaana Chakra

English Name:

The Sacral Chakra

Symbol:
Crescent moon within A Lotus with 6 petals.

Colour:
Orange/Vermilion

Location:
Sacrum. (Lower Abdomen region)

Element:
Water.

Glands it Controls:
Sexual glands. (Testes and the Ovaries)

Organs it Controls:
Organs from the lower abdomen region, mainly the reproductive organs.

Food that nourishes this Chakra:
Milk and dairy products, Melons, Bananas, Honey, Chocolate, Butter and Red Wine in Moderation.

The Sacral Chakra is located on the spine at the sacral level, hence the name. It is associated and responsible for the health of the sexual organs and Urinary system. When this Chakra is balanced, you will feel free and joyous and you will exude an amazing sexual confidence.

Mudras for Awakening & Balancing Svadhishtaana / The Sacral Chakra

While performing these Mudras, Concentrate on your breathing and visualize a ray of bright Orange light entering your Sacral Chakra and the Chakra glowing in a bright Orange Luminescence.

SvadhishtaanaChakramudra / Mudra of Pelvic Centre Chakra

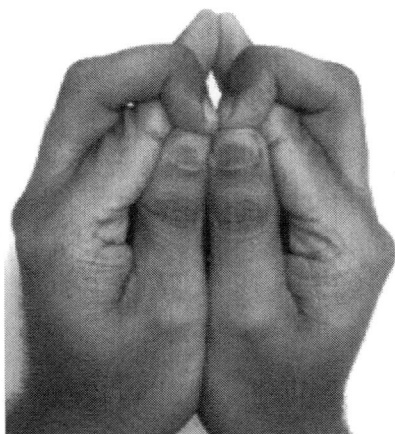

Method:

This Mudra can be performed while being seated, in a standing position or lying in bed.

Concentrate on your breathing to relax and feel comfortable.

Join both the palms together like in the Indian salutation 'Namaste'.

Then interlace and bend the Ring fingers and the Little fingers of both the hands within the palms.

Cross the Middle fingers over the Index fingers.

Touch the tip of the Middle fingers to the tip of the Thumbs and press slightly.

Press the heels of both the palms together.

Hold this Mudra in front of your chest.

Duration:

This Mudra should be performed for at least 5 minutes and can be performed for 40 minutes at a stretch.

This Mudra should be performed twice a day, once in the morning and once in the evening for best results.

Shaktimudra / Mudra of Divine Feminine

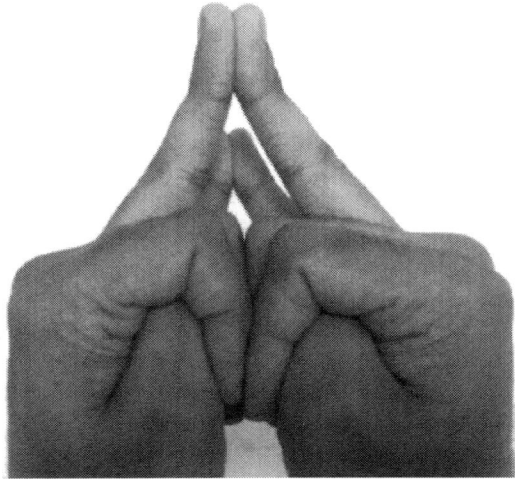

Method:

This Mudra has to be performed in a seating position.

Be seated comfortably in an upright posture and concentrate on your breathing to relax.

Keep your palms facing each other in front of your chest.

Then touch the tips of both your Little fingers and press slightly.

Mudras for Awakening Chakras

After that, touch the tips of both your Ring fingers and press slightly.

Fold your thumbs in to your palms

And, cover up the folded thumbs curling down your Index and Middle fingers into your palms.

Duration:

This Mudra should be performed for at least 5 minutes and can be performed for 40 minutes at a stretch.

This Mudra should be performed twice a day, once in the morning and once in the evening for best results.

Kaamjayimudra / Mudra to Conquer Lust

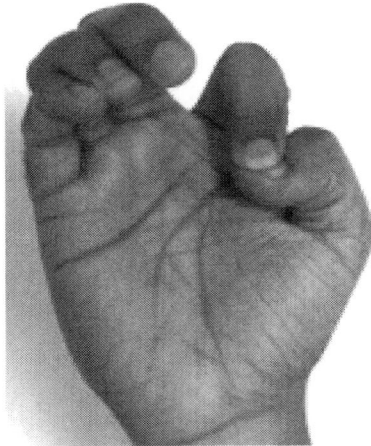

Method:

This Mudra can be performed while being seated, in a standing position or lying in bed.

Concentrate on your breathing to relax and feel comfortable.

Touch the tip of the Index finger to the nail of your Thumb and press slightly.

Curl down the remaining three fingers, and press them together (not too tight).

Refer to the image for more clarity.

Duration:

This Mudra does not have a specific duration; it should be performed till the desired results are achieved.

*Note

The Kaamjayi Mudra was used by ancient Indian Maharshi's and Yogi's to suppress their sexual desires.

**Important

Don't overdo this Mudra, you sexual desires are a healthy part of your relationships. There's nothing to feel guilty about your sexual desires.

Manipur Chakra / The Abdominal Chakra (The Solar Plexus Chakra)

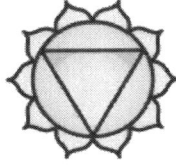

Sanskrit Name:

मणिपूर चक्र - Manipur Chakra

English Name:

The Abdominal Chakra / The Solar Plexus Chakra.

Symbol:
Downward pointing triangle within A Lotus with 10 petals.

Colour:
Yellow

Location:
Solar Plexus. (Just beneath the Diaphragm)

Element:
Fire. (Since it is related to digestion)

Glands it Controls:
Adrenal Glands and the Pancreas.

Organs it Controls:
Organs of the digestive system.

Food that nourishes this Chakra:
Fish, Chicken, Eggs, Oranges, Papaya, Apricots, Carrots.

The Solar Plexus Chakra is located on the spine at a level just beneath the diaphragm, hence the name. It is associated and responsible for the health of Stomach, Liver, Pancreas and the Spleen. When this Chakra is balanced, you will feel satisfied and an affectionate adoration towards your loved ones and it induces a feeling of being in control.

Mudras for Awakening & Balancing Manipur / The Abdominal Chakra

While performing these Mudras, Concentrate on your breathing and visualize a ray of bright Yellow light entering your Abdominal Chakra and the Chakra glowing in a bright Yellow Luminescence.

ManipurChakramudra / Mudra of Solar Plexus Chakra

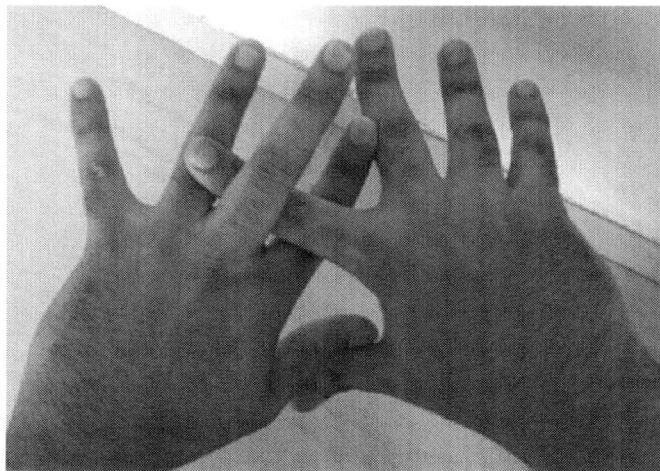

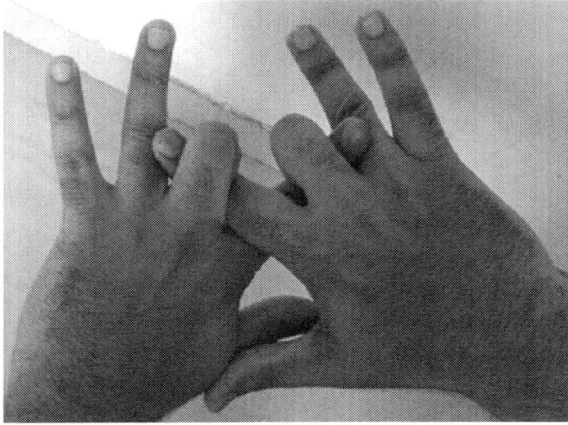

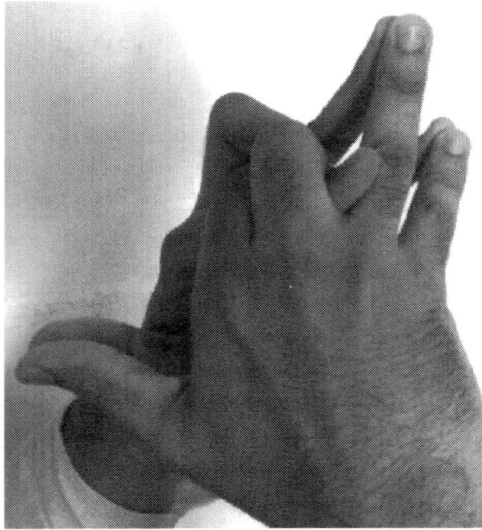

Method:

This Mudra has to be performed in a seating position.

Mudras for Awakening Chakras

Be seated comfortably in an upright posture and concentrate on your breathing to relax.

Place your palms adjacent to each other, facing down.

Now slide your right Index finger over your left Index finger, then under the left Middle finger and then rest it over the left Ring finger. (I know it sounds very confusing, please refer the adjoining images for more clarity.)

Now curl in your left Middle finger, pressing the down the right Index finger.

The next step is to curl in the right middle finger so that it presses down the left Index finger, but see to it that the tip of the left Index finger is over the right Ring finger. (refer the image)

Now join the tips of both the Ring and Little fingers together and press slightly.

Then join the tips of both the Thumbs together and press slightly.

Hold the Mudra in front of your solar plexus.

Duration:

This Mudra should be performed for at least 5 minutes and can be performed for 30 minutes at a stretch.

This Mudra should be performed twice a day, once in the morning and once in the evening for best results.

Rudramudra / Mudra of Lord Shiva

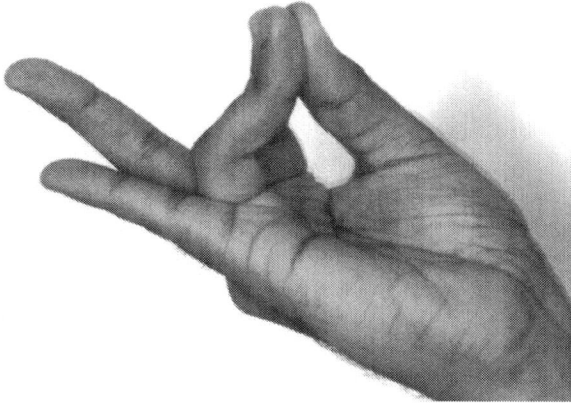

Method:

This Mudra has to be performed in a seating position.

Be seated comfortably in an upright posture and concentrate on your breathing to relax.

Place your hands on your thighs with your palms facing upwards.

Touch the tip of your Thumb with the tip of your Index finger and the tip of the Ring finger, press slightly.

Refer the image for more clarity.

Duration:

This Mudra should be performed for at least 5 minutes and can be performed for 40 minutes at a stretch.

If you are serious about losing weight then this Mudra should be performed at least 4 times a day.

Adhomukhmudra / Mudra that Faces Down

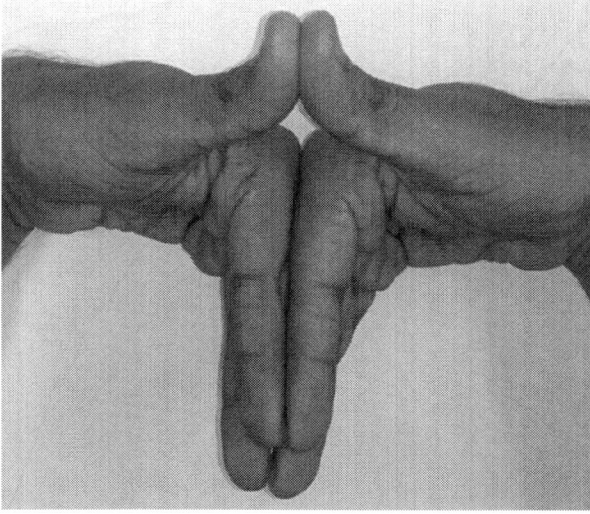

Method:

This Mudra has to be performed in a seating position.

Be seated comfortably in an upright posture and concentrate on your breathing to relax.

Now bring both your palms in front of you, the palms should be facing downward.

Join the tips of both your Thumbs and press slightly.

All other fingers should be pointed downwards and outstretched in such a way that all the nails are resting on each other. (refer the image)

Duration:

It's a highly effective Mudra, also a very strong one.

Perform this Mudra for not more than 5-7 minutes at a time, and a t total of 3-4 sessions per day.

Garudamudra / Mudra of Eagle

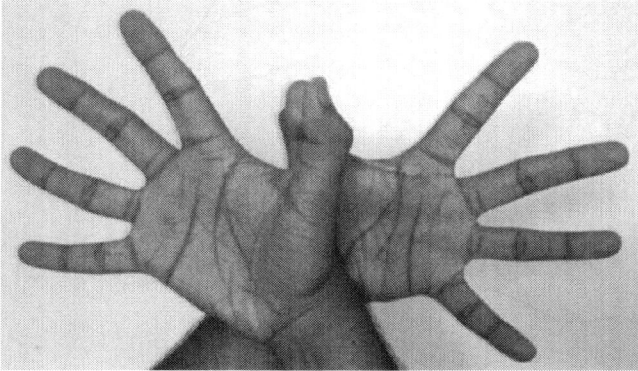

Method:

This Mudra can be performed while being seated, in a standing position or lying in bed.

Concentrate on your breathing to relax and feel comfortable.

Bring both your hands in front of your chest, palms facing the chest.

Cross the hands with the right hand crossing over the left hand and interlock the Thumbs at the first padding. (Refer the image)

Keep all the other fingers extended and outstretched.

Create a firm pressure between the pads of the
Thumb.

Duration:

This Mudra should be performed for at least 5
minutes and can be performed for 40 minutes at a
stretch.

This Mudra should be performed twice a day,
once in the morning and once in the evening for
best results.

Surabhimudra (Dhenumudra) / Mudra of Cow

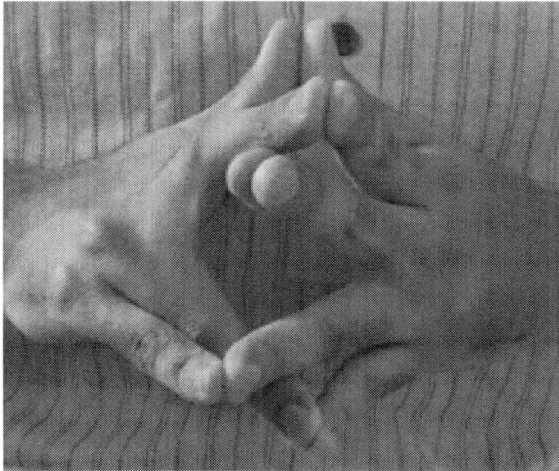

Method:

This Mudra has to be performed in a seating position.

Be seated comfortably in an upright posture and concentrate on your breathing to relax.

Touch the tip of the Little finger of the left hand to the tip of the Ring finger of the right hand.

Touch the tip of the Middle finger of the left hand to the tip of the Index finger of the right hand.

Touch the tip of the ring finger of the left hand to the tip of the Little finger of the right hand.

Touch the tip of the Index finger of the left hand to the tip of the Middle finger of the right hand. (This is a bit confusing; refer to the image for clarity)

Then join the tips of both the Thumbs together and press slightly.

Hold this Mudra in front of your chest.

Duration:

This Mudra should be performed for at least 5 minutes and can be performed for 30 minutes at a stretch.

This Mudra should be performed twice a day, once in the morning and once in the evening for best results.

Anaahat Chakra / The Heart Chakra

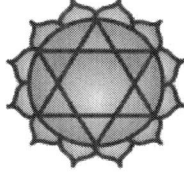

Sanskrit Name:

अनाहत चक्र - Anaahat Chakra

English Name:

The Heart Chakra

Symbol:
Six pointed star within a Circular flower with 12 petals.

Colour:
Green.

Location:
Chest.

Element:
Air.

Glands it Controls:
The Thymus Gland. (It is responsible for a sound Immune system.)

Organs it Controls:
Heart, Lungs, Upper limbs, Organs of the Circulatory system and Immune system.

Food that nourishes this Chakra:
Cherries, Strawberries, Whole Wheat, Unpolished Rice, Soya bean, Green Leafy Vegetables (especially Spinach).

The Heart Chakra is located on the spine at the level of the Heart, hence the name. It is associated and responsible for the cardiovascular health and the health of the respiratory system and also keeps the immune system healthy. On an emotional level this Chakra is about affection, love, care and romance. This Chakra enables one to give and receive pure love.

Mudras for Awakening & Balancing Anaahat Chakra / The Heart Chakra

While performing these Mudras, Concentrate on your breathing and visualize a ray of bright Green light entering your Heart Chakra and the Chakra glowing in a bright Green Luminescence.

AnaahatChakramudra / Mudra of Unstruck Hymn

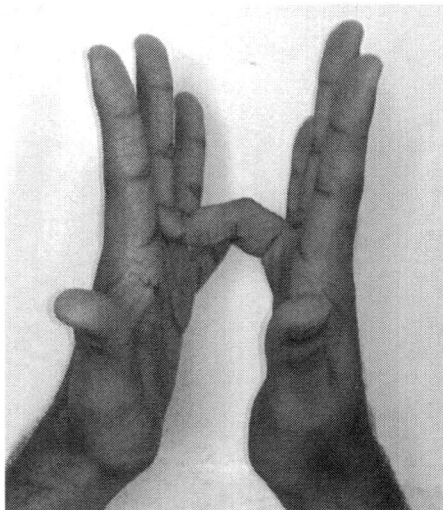

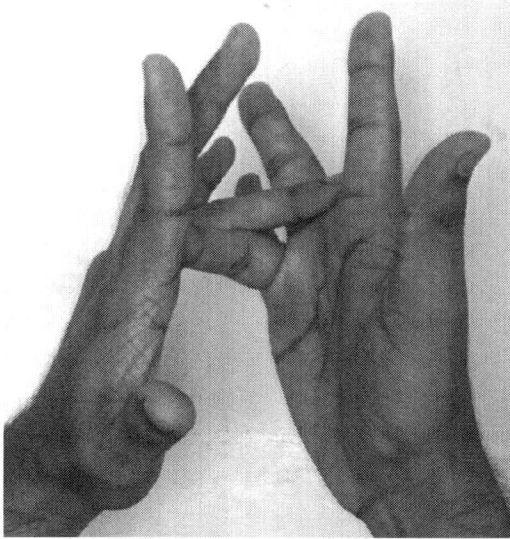

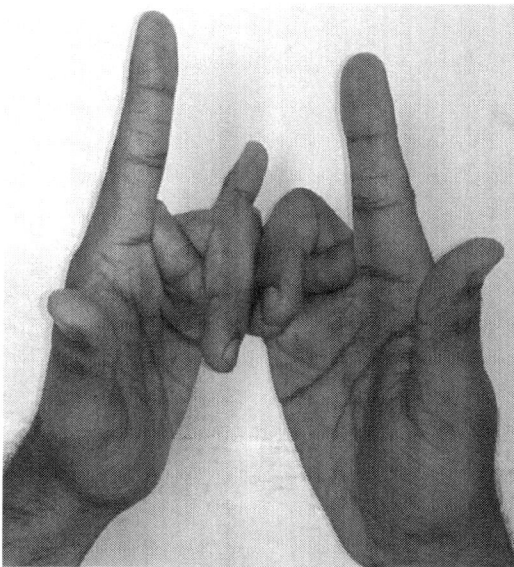

Advait

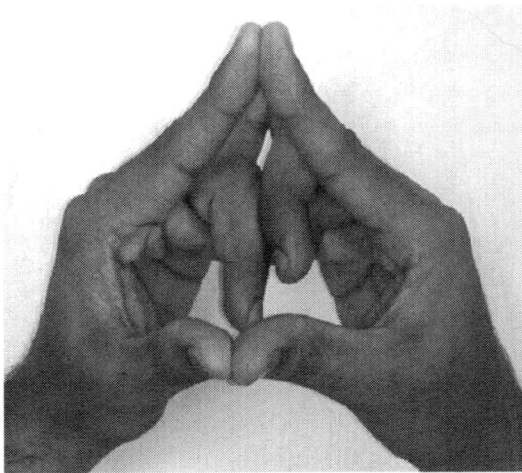

Method:

This Mudra has to be performed in a seating position.

Be seated comfortably in an upright posture and concentrate on your breathing to relax.

Place the right Ring finger on the web between the Index and Middle finger of the left hand.

Place the left Ring finger on the web between the Index and Middle finger of the right hand.

Curl down both the middle fingers to wrap and press down the respective Ring fingers of the opposite hands.

Now join the tips of both the Index and Little fingers together, outstretch them and press slightly.

Then join the tips of both the Thumbs together, outstretch them and press slightly.

This Mudra is to be held in front of your chest.

Duration:

This Mudra should be performed for at least 5 minutes and can be performed for 40 minutes at a stretch.

This Mudra should be performed twice a day, once in the morning and once in the evening for best results.

Padmamudra (Pankajmudra) / Mudra of Lotus

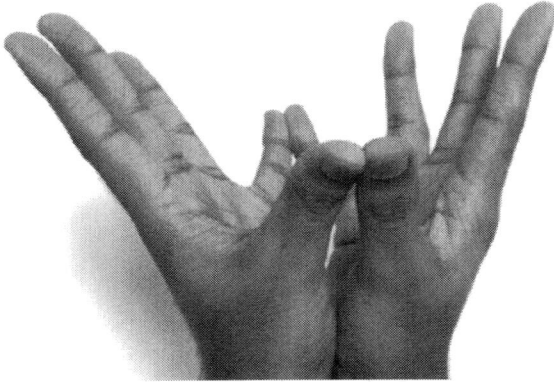

Method:

This Mudra has to be performed in a seating position.

Be seated comfortably in an upright posture and concentrate on your breathing to relax.

Touch the Thumb and Little finger of the left hand to the Thumb and Little finger of the right hand.

Join the base of both the palms together.

Stretch all the other fingers outwards and keep them straight.

Refer the image above.

This Mudra should be held in front of your chest.

Duration:

This Mudra should be performed for at least 5 minutes and can be performed for 40 minutes at a stretch.

This Mudra should be performed twice a day, once in the morning and once in the evening for best results.

Mrutsanjivanimudra
(Apaanvaayumudra) / Mudra of Resurrection

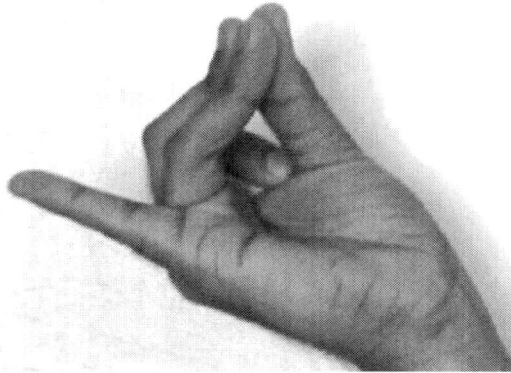

Method:

This Mudra has to be performed in a seating position.

Be seated comfortably in an upright posture and concentrate on your breathing to relax.

Touch the base of your Thumb with the tip of the Index finger and press slightly.

Then, touch the tips of the Index finger, Middle finger and Thumb together.

Keep the Little finger extended outwards.

Perform the Mudra's on both your hands and place them on your thighs.

Duration:

This Mudra should be performed for at least 5 minutes and can be performed for 40 minutes at a stretch.

This Mudra should be performed twice a day, once in the morning and once in the evening for best results.

Vishuddha Chakra / The Throat Chakra

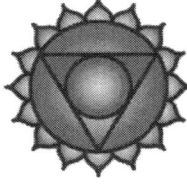

Sanskrit Name:

वशिुद्ध चक्र - Vishuddha Chakra (Vishuddhi = Purification)

English Name:

The Throat Chakra / The Chakra of Purification

Symbol:
A Circle housed within a downward facing Triangle, which is housed in a flower with 16 petals.

Colour:
Blue / Turquoise

Location:
Throat.

Element:
Sound. (The base element is 'Air', since air when modulated creates sound)

Glands it Controls:
Thyroid

Organs it Controls:
Throat, Neck and other Oral organs.

Food that nourishes this Chakra:
Mushrooms, Bananas, Kelp, Wheat Grass juice.

The Throat Chakra is located on the spine along the throat, hence the name. It is associated and responsible for the health of the Throat, Neck and the Thyroid Gland. When this Chakra is balanced, it induces proper growth and you will feel aware about the people around you and you will feel active creatively.

Mudras for Awakening & Balancing Vishuddha Chakra / The Throat Chakra

While performing these Mudras, Concentrate on your breathing and visualize a ray of bright Blue light entering your Throat Chakra and the Chakra glowing in a bright Blue Luminescence.

VishuddhaChakramudra / Mudra of Throat Chakra

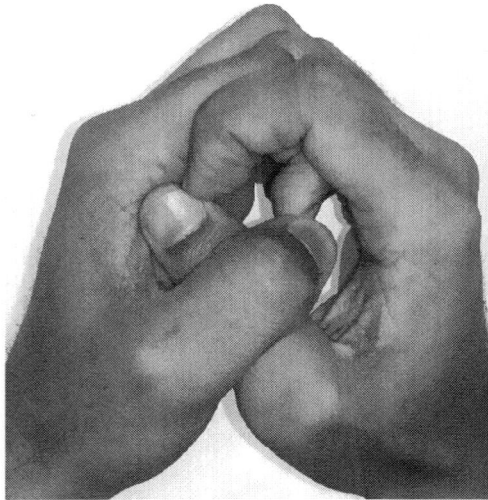

Method:

This Mudra has to be performed in a seating position.

Be seated comfortably in an upright posture and concentrate on your breathing to relax.

Join the hands together as in the Indian salutation, 'Namaste'.

Now, interlace the Middle, Ring and Little into the palm (Refer the image)

Then, create two interlocking rings with the Index fingers and Thumbs as shown in the image.

Hold this Mudra in front of your Throat.

Duration:

This Mudra should be performed for at least 5 minutes and can be performed for 40 minutes at a stretch.

This Mudra should be performed twice a day, once in the morning and once in the evening for best results.

Granthitamudra / Mudra of Glands

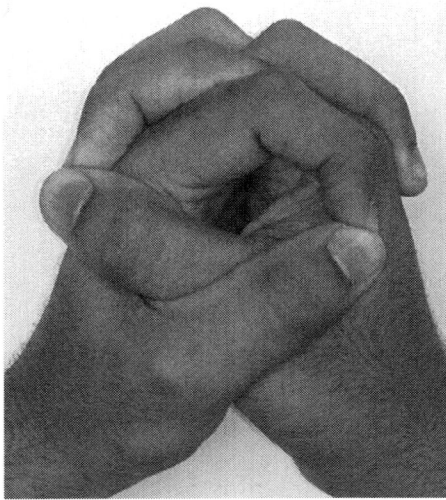

Method:

This Mudra has to be performed in a seating position.

Be seated comfortably in an upright posture and concentrate on your breathing to relax.

Clasp both your hands together as shown in the image.

Note that the left index figure is on top of the right index finger.

Now, join the tips of the Index finger and Thumb of the respective hands together.

Hold this Mudra in front of your Throat.

Duration:

This Mudra should be performed for at least 5 minutes and can be performed for 40 minutes at a stretch.

This Mudra should be performed twice a day, once in the morning and once in the evening for best results.

Aadnya (Ajna) Chakra / The Third Eye Chakra

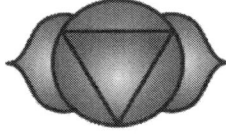

Sanskrit Name:

आज्ञा चक्र - Aadnya Chakra

English Name:

The Third Eye Chakra

Symbol:
A Lotus with two petals.

Colour:
Violet / Indigo.

Location:
Half a centimeter above the midpoint between the two eyebrows.

Element:
Light.

Glands it Controls:
Pineal Glands.

Organs it Controls:
Eyes, Ears, Nose and Brain.

Food that nourishes this Chakra:
Wheat, food stuffs rich in Vitamin E and Vitamin A, Sprouts.

The Third Eye Chakra is located at the point of the third eye, hence the name. It is associated and responsible for the health of the eyes and the entire nervous system. When this Chakra is balanced, you will feel an insightful awareness and also feel very clairvoyant.

Mudras for Awakening & Balancing Aadnya Chakra / The Third Eye Chakra

While performing these Mudras, Concentrate on your breathing and visualize a ray of bright Indigo light entering your Third-Eye Chakra and the Chakra glowing in a bright Indigo Luminescence.

Nirvaanamudra / Mudra of Liberation

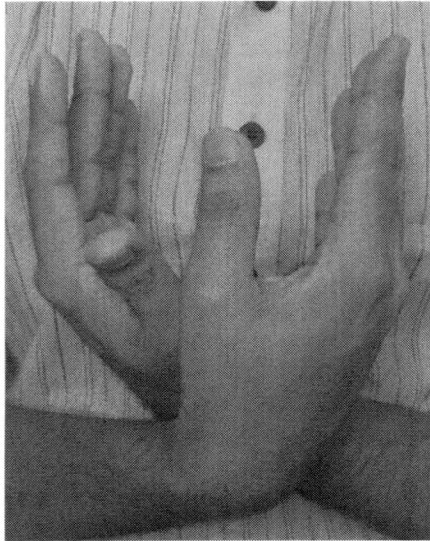

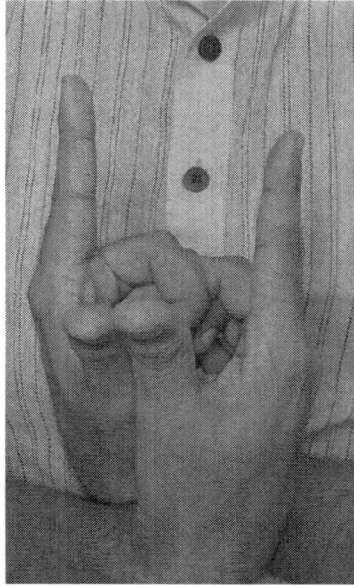

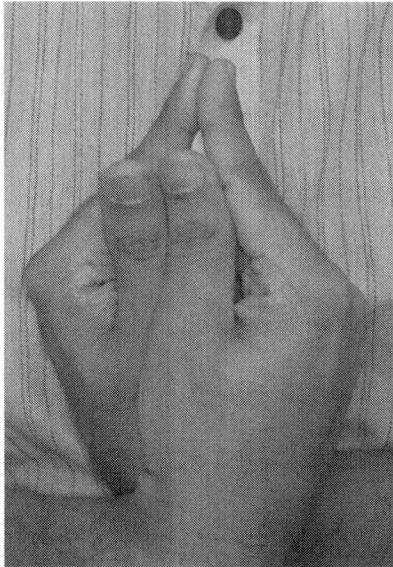

Advait

Method:

This Mudra has to be performed in a seating position.

Be seated comfortably in an upright posture and concentrate on your breathing to relax.

Cross your hands at your wrists in front of your face, with your left hand crossing over the right hand.

Now, fold/curl down the Little, Ring and Middle fingers of both the hands.

Now, touch the tips of both the Index fingers together, while keeping your Thumbs parallel to each other and touching.

Then, gently bow down your head and let the tip of the index fingers touch the Third-Eye point. (The Third-Eye point is located half a centimeter above the midpoint between the eyebrows.)

Hold for 1 to 2 minutes.

While performing this Mudra visualize your third eye opening and wherever you see, there is peace and calmness.

Duration:

1 to 2 minutes.

Mahashirshamudra / Mudra of The Great Head

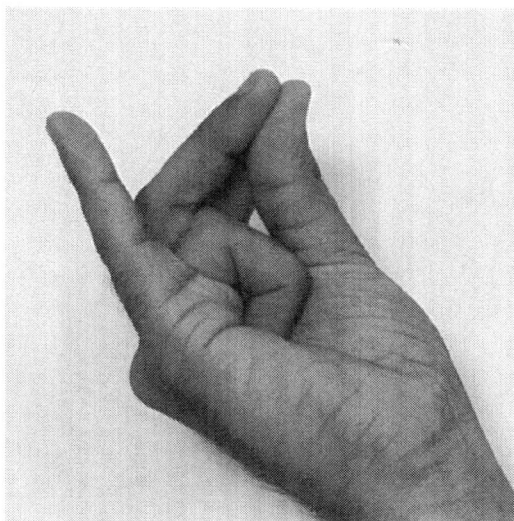

Method:

This Mudra has to be performed in a seating position.

Be seated comfortably in an upright posture and concentrate on your breathing to relax.

Touch the centre of the palm with the tip of the Ring finger.

Join the tips of the Index finger, Middle finger and Thumb together.

Keep the Little finger extended outwards.

(Refer the image)

Perform this Mudra on each hand and place the hands in your lap.

Duration:

This Mudra should be performed for at least 5 minutes and can be performed for 20 minutes at a stretch.

This Mudra should be performed twice a day, once in the morning and once in the evening for best results.

Sahastraar Chakra / The Crown Chakra

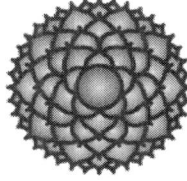

Sanskrit Name:

सहस्रार चक्र - Sahastraar Chakra (Sahastraar = A Thousand Petals)

English Name:

The Crown Chakra

Symbol:
A Lotus with Thousand petals.

Colour:
Multicolored or sometimes White.

Location:
Just above the Crown of the skull.

Element:
Space.

Glands it Controls:

The Entire Central Nervous system.

Organs it Controls:
Cerebrum, Spinal Cord and Organs of the Nervous System.

The Crown Chakra is located on the crown of the skull, hence the name. It is associated and responsible for the health of the pineal glands and the nervous system. When this Chakra is balanced, you will feel extremely satisfied and blissful. It is the most spiritual Chakra.

Mudras for Awakening & Balancing Sahastraar Chakra / The Crown Chakra

While performing these Mudras, Concentrate on your breathing and visualize a ray of bright White light entering your Crown Chakra and the Chakra glowing in a bright White Luminescence.

Sahastraarmudra / Mudra of Thousand Petals

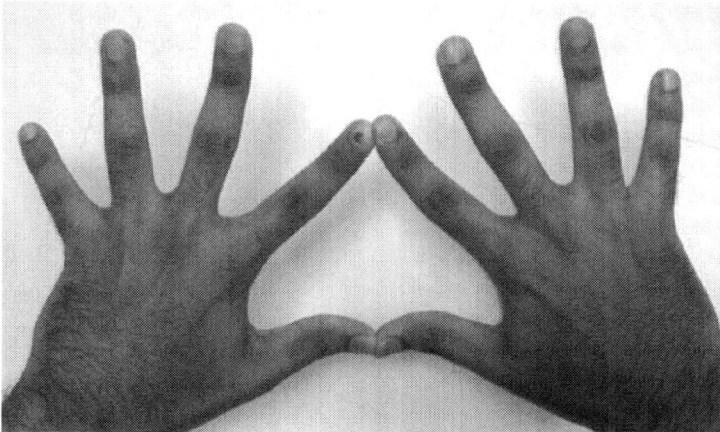

Method:

This Mudra can be performed while being seated, in a standing position.

Concentrate on your breathing to relax and feel comfortable.

Raise your hands at chest height, with your palms facing down.

Now, join the tips of both the Index fingers together and press slightly.

Then, join the tips of both the Thumbs together forming a Triangle. (Refer the image)

Keep all the other fingers extended and outstretched.

Once you have formed this Mudra, raise the Mudra at a height of around 6 inches above your head.

And now visualize as if a shower of light and energy are entering the top of your head through the triangle formed in the Mudra.

Duration:

This Mudra should be performed for at least 5 minutes and can be performed for 20 minutes at a stretch.

This Mudra should be performed twice a day, once in the morning and once in the evening for best results.

Forming a Routine

Every Mudra that I have mentioned in this book has to be performed for at least five minutes for best results.

But, to perform all the 19 Mudras for at least 5 minutes will eat up a little over 1 and a 1/2 hrs of your time every day and many of you might not be able to take off that much time every day from your busy schedules and chores.

Understand that it is NOT a hard and fast rule that you should perform all these 19 Mudras back to back in one session.

What I would suggest is, perform any one (1) Mudra pertaining to each of the seven Chakras daily. Thus, you'll have to take out only a minimum of 35 minutes every day.

(Make sure that you perform all the 19 Mudras at least thrice in a week.)

The beauty of Mudra Health and Healing Techniques is that Mudras can be performed at any time and place: while stuck in traffic, at the office, watching TV, or whenever you have to twiddle your thumbs waiting for something or someone.

So, please don't come up with any excuses to avoid them, Mudras are as Easy and Effortless as Chakra Awakening and Balancing could get.

Free 7 Day email course

"Sukshma Asanas for Awakening Chakras"

The Mudras in themselves are a very effective technique for Chakra Awakening. But, do you know that you can increase the effectiveness of these Mudras, manifolds?

Let me explain how...

Yogic philosophy puts a lot of emphasis on the concept of Action (karm) and Inaction (akarm).

These concepts have great philosophical as well as physical implications.

On a physical level, according to yoga, action followed by inaction gives greater and far more effective results.

'Action' acts as a *stimulant* and then 'Inaction' acts as a *re-enforcement*.

In this case,

Mudras represent inaction, and when you perform certain micro-exercises called as "Sukshma Asanas", which represent action, before practicing the Mudras, the effect and intensity of Mudras increase exponentially.

In simple terms; performing sukshma asanas before practicing the Mudras works wonders.

I have compiled 7 such sukshma asanas, one for each chakra, into a 7 day email course.

And, I am offering the online email course, for **FREE** to my readers only.

Get your Free 7 day email course; **"Sukshma Asanas for Awakening Chakras"** here:

https://goo.gl/nRWLb

Simply type the link in your web browser to get the free email course and fast track your Chakra Awakening process.

-Advait

Other books on Mudras by Advait

P.S. All my books are enrolled in the 'Kindle Unlimited Program' you can read all of my books for free through **'Kindle Unlimited'**.

- - -

Mudras for Spiritual Healing: 21 Simple Hand Gestures for Ultimate Spiritual Healing & Awakening

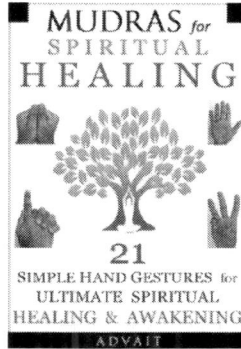

http://www.amazon.com/dp/B00PFYZLQO

Mudras: 25 Ultimate techniques for Self Healing

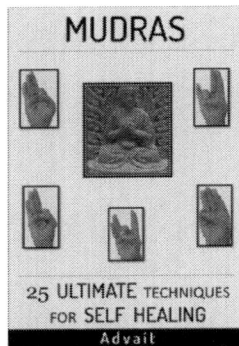

http://www.amazon.com/dp/B00MMPB5CI

Mudras for Awakening Chakras

Mudras for Sex: 25 Simple Hand Gestures for Extreme Erotic Pleasure & Sexual Vitality

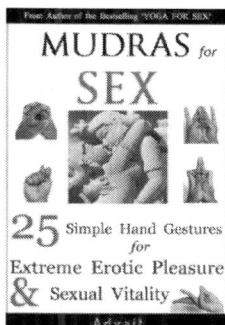

http://www.amazon.com/dp/B00OJR1DRY

Mudras for Weight Loss: 21 Simple Hand Gestures for Effortless Weight Loss

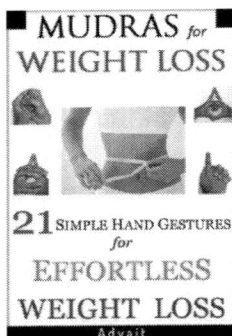

http://www.amazon.com/dp/B00P3ZPSEK

Mudras for a Strong Heart: 21 Simple Hand Gestures for Preventing, Curing & Reversing Heart Disease

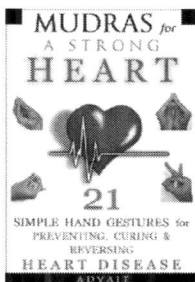

http://www.amazon.com/dp/B00PFRLGTM

Mudras for Curing Cancer: 21 Simple Hand
Gestures for Preventing & Curing Cancer

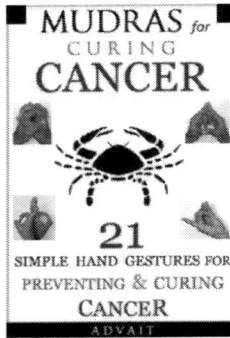

http://www.amazon.com/dp/B00PFO199M

Mudras for Anxiety: 25 Simple Hand Gestures for Curing Your Anxiety

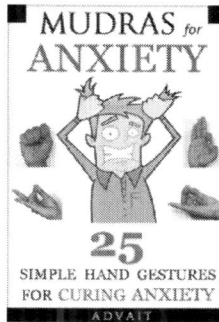

http://www.amazon.com/dp/B00PF011IU

Mudras for Stress Management: 21 Simple Hand
Gestures for a Stress Free Life

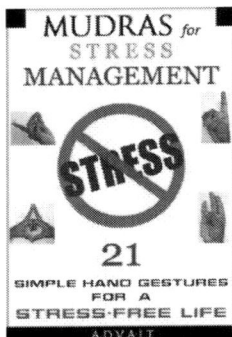

http://amazon.com/dp/B00PFTJ6OC

Mudras for Awakening Chakras

Mudras for Memory Improvement: 25 Simple Hand Gestures for Ultimate Memory Improvement

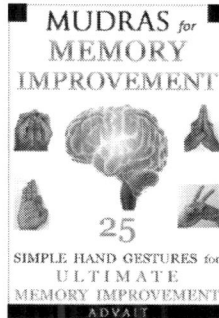

http://www.amazon.com/dp/B00PFSP8TK

Thank You

Thank you so much for reading my book. I hope you really liked it.

As you probably know, many people look at the reviews on Amazon before they decide to purchase a book.

If you liked the book, please take a minute to leave a review with your feedback.

60 seconds is all I'm asking for, and it would mean a lot to me.

Thank You so much.

All the best,

Advait

Other Books by Advait

Yoga for Sex: 30 Simple Exercises for Ultimate
Sexual Pleasure

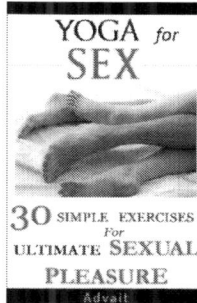

http://www.amazon.com/dp/B00OAXI8R0

Ayurveda of Diet: 15 Ultimate Eating Habits
Recommended in Ayurveda for Health and
Healing

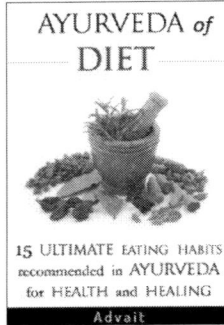

Mudras for Awakening Chakras

Ayurveda of Garlic: 25 Ultimate uses of Garlic for Health and Healing

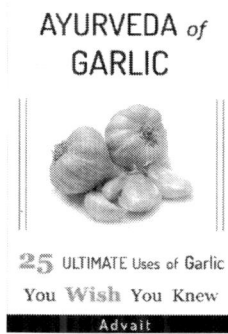

http://www.amazon.com/dp/B00N8YKTLU

On Ancient Teaching Techniques

Vedic Mathematics – Multiplication Made Easy:
Learn to Multiply 25 times Faster in a Day!!

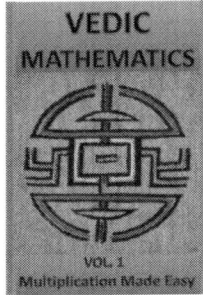

http://www.amazon.com/dp/B00I3LDWAI

On Ancient Feng Shui Techniques

Feng Shui for Wealth: 20 Ultimate Accessories for Attracting Wealth and How to Use Them.

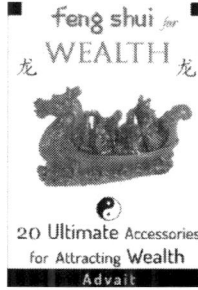

http://www.amazon.com/dp/B00NI7GCPY

Books on Yoga

Easy Yoga: Your Ultimate Beginners Guide to
Understanding Yoga and Leading a Disease-Free
Life through Routine Yoga Practice

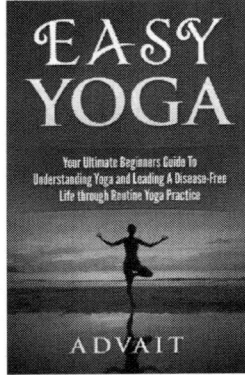

http://www.amazon.com/dp/B010I97366

Monday Yoga: Pranayam and Sukshma-Asanas for starting Your Routine Yoga Practice and Inducing Vigor into Your Life on the first day of the Week

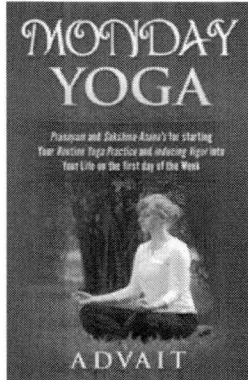

http://www.amazon.com/dp/B011SI6MK4

Tuesday Yoga: 12 Yoga Asanas to be performed on Tuesday as a Part of Your Daily Yoga Routine

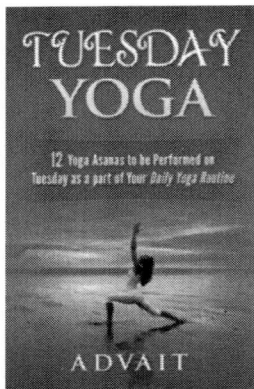

http://www.amazon.com/dp/B013GGA1AS

Wednesday Yoga: 12 Yoga Asanas to be performed on Wednesday as a Part of Your Daily Yoga Routine

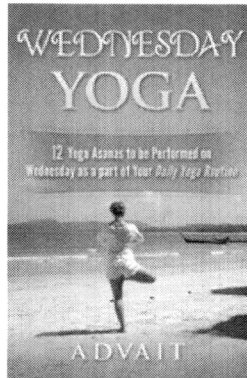

http://www.amazon.com/dp/B014RTDQ5U

Thursday Yoga: 12 Yoga Asanas to be performed on Thursday as a Part of Your Daily Yoga Routine

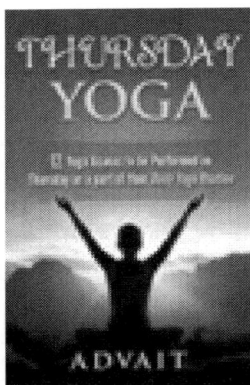

http://www.amazon.com/dp/B015JMSEPQ

Mudras for Awakening Chakras

Friday Yoga: 12 Yoga Asanas to be performed on
Friday as a Part of Your Daily Yoga Routine

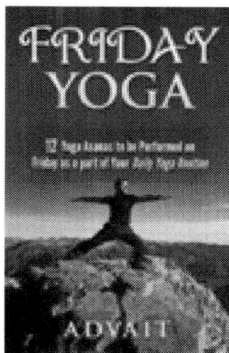

http://www.amazon.com/dp/B015UK17KG

Book Excerpt

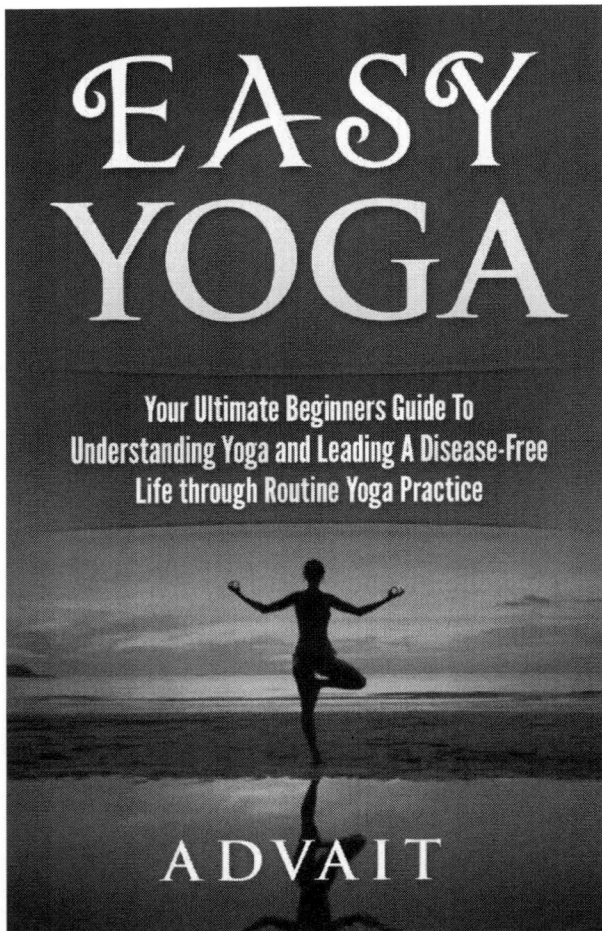

Mudras for Awakening Chakras

'Easy Yoga'

*Your Ultimate Beginners Guide
to Understanding Yoga and
Leading a Disease-Free Life
through Routine Yoga Practice*

Advait

Contents

Mudras for Awakening Chakras

Disclaimer and FTC Notice

The True Meaning of Yoga

There is a common and popular belief that 'Yoga' is an Indian ritual which is all about performing difficult physical exercises for maintaining health and curing diseases.

This is a MYTH!!

Actually, Sound Health is a side-effect of Yoga.

Surprising!!! But true.

The word 'Yoga' literally means *to unite ourselves with our higher self* - an entirely meta-physical objective which can be achieved through a Discipline of Physical exercises (Asana's) coupled with Meditation exercises (*Dhyana*) and Breathing exercises (Pranayam). When we perform those exercises we get in shape and achieve good health.

Yoga is not something to be performed or practiced, it is to be achieved.

Yoga is the destination and the path to it is through a disciplined practice of physical exercises, meditation and breathing exercises.

Maharshi Patanjali, in his revolutionary work *'Paatanjal YogaSutra'* prescribes an eight-fold path to achieve Yoga, known as *Ashtang Yoga*.

['Paatanjal YogaSutra' is considered to be the most comprehensive book on Yoga and it forms the basis and reference of all the Yoga methodologies practiced throughout the world today.]

The Ashtang Yoga [eight-fold path to yoga], given by Maharshi Patanjali is as follows:

Yama

The moral virtues that one should possess as they are considered to be essential for one's initiation on the path to yoga.

Niyama

It involves being knowledgeable and aware about your surroundings and then studying your-self to form an essential discipline which you would adhere to.

Asana

Understanding and Performing the required physical exercises, this is the core of your yoga practice.

Pranayam

It is all about breath control, which enhances the life energy which governs the existence of a being and balances the mental energy.

Pratyahar

Sensory inhibitions which internalize the consciousness and prepare your mind to take action.

Dharana

It involves inculcating an extended mental focus to concentrate on only those things that are essential.

Dhyana

It involves meditation, paying attention to your breathing and thus focusing only on yourself.

Samadhi

Becoming one with the object of your contemplation and experiencing spiritual liberation.

Yama and Niyama are essential for inculcating the needed discipline and establish a strict routine.

Asana is the crucial physical part, which subjects your body to essential physical movements through different exercises.

Pranayam and Pratyahar are needed to guide us through the various breathing exercises and for making us aware of the internal spiritual changes as we ascend along the path to Yoga.

Dharana and Dhyana stages prepare us mentally and spiritually to concentrate inwards by using various meditation exercises.

Samadhi is the culmination stage where one achieves Yoga.

A Brief History of Yoga

Before going any further let's look back at where it all began.

To tell you the truth.... No one knows!!

The foundation of Yoga as a science is attributed to *Maharshi Patanjali* who lived in India in 3rd Century B.C.

But, archeological excavations in the Indus Valley civilization sites have unearthed sculptures and idols depicting various Asana's (physical exercise positions) suggested in Yoga and these idols date back to around 3000 years B.C.

Also, information about various aspects of Yoga can be found in Vedic texts like; Shwetashwatrupanishad,

Chaandogyopanishad,

Kaushitki Upanishad,

Maitri Upanishad etc.

This information was scattered all over and Maharshi Patanjali, compiled these nuggets into a streamlined and strict science of Yoga or should I say he compiled this scattered information into a way of life called *Yoga* through his work 'Paatanjal YogaSutra'

After Maharshi Patanjali,

Maharshi Swatwaram wrote 'Hatapradipika' (meaning - One Which Illuminates the Path of Hatha Yoga , i.e. the physical aspect of Yoga) in the 13th Century A.D.

And, Maharshi Gherand wrote 'Gherandsanhita' around the same time.

Almost all the Yoga methodologies practiced world-over today regard Maharshi Patanjali's work as their reference.

Importance of a *Yoga Routine*

I like to keep all my books absolutely fluff free and concise. I promise you, this book will be no different.

I will not waste 10 pages in convincing you about how amazing Yoga is and how you can benefit from practicing it. But, I will tell you this...

If you want to live at least a **100 years of disease-free life** *and want the same for your loved ones, the only thing that can guarantee it is a Yoga Routine.*

Many western scholars claim that Ancient Indian Seer's (Maharshi's) had a life span of well over a century and they attribute this longevity to a regular practice of Yoga by these Maharshi's.

For e.g.: Maharshi Vyaas, is attributed to compiling and categorizing the scattered Vedic Knowledge and Wisdom into the four Veda's (that's the reason why is also called as Maharshi Ved Vyaas), he is also attributed for writing 'Mahabharata' (mind you, the 'Bhagavad Gita' is but a small part of Mahabharata) and numerous other works, and many scholars and historians have concluded that it is not possible to do all this in an average life span of 60-70 years, so he had to have lived well over a century.

Such similar comparisons can also be drawn true to numerous other Philosophers, Thinkers and Acharya's of Vedic India.

The bottom-line is, a well established, sincere and disciplined *Yoga Routine* is the best medical insurance you can have for yourself and your family.

Types of Yoga Exercises

It is impossible to make a general classification of Yoga Asana's (exercises), as each Asana can be classified into multiple sub-categories, for e.g.;

A. Asana's can be classified depending upon whether you hold your breath in while performing the exercise, you exhale and perform the exercise or you maintain your normal rate of breathing.

B. Asana's can be classified depending upon whether you perform it standing, sitting or lying down on the mat.

C. Asana's can also be classified depending upon the parts of the body being extended and stretched.

For our ease and understanding, in this book and in the subsequent 'Yoga Routine' series, we broadly classify Asana's into Three (3) categories:

I. Dhyanasana's:

Asana's which don't involve much physical movement, but focus more on mental focus and concentration, with a hint of meditation, viz. *Swastikasan.*

II. Vyayamasana's: (vyayam = physical exercise)

Asana's which mainly focus on physical movements and stretching, viz. *Taulasan.*

III. Vishrantiasana's: (Vishranti = Rest/Relaxation)

Asana's which are used to relax and rest your body after performing physical Asana's, viz. *Shavasan.*

Some Essential Precautions

Here are some precautions and rules you need to follow if you wish to achieve best results;

1. Yoga is very helpful if done in the Morning and on an empty stomach (don't eat anything, you can drink water). If you cannot make time in the morning, you can practice it in the evening but make sure that you practice it after 4 to 4 ½ Hrs. of having your meals.

2. When you get up in the morning , have a glass of water, visit the toilet (what I mean is, take a poop), take a shower and then do Yoga, as water will rejuvenate your system and taking a shower will warm up your body for the exercises you are about to perform.

3. Understand this; You are the only essential for Yoga and not your clothes. I find all the recent 'yoga attire' fad to be pointless. All you need is a simple mat to sit on, A Pajama and a loose T-shirt which don't restrict your movements while you perform the Asana's.

4. Take your time while performing the Asana's, don't hurry through the exercises as if you are on a deadline. Remember, 'Yoga is for You...You are not for Yoga'. If you find yourself short on time,

don't perform all the listed exercises in a hurry, practice only a few that you can in that short time, but slowly and steadily.

5. Don't let your mind wander off while doing the Asana's, concentrate on your movements instead. A very easy trick is to concentrate on your breathing.

6. Women should not perform Yoga during menstruation.

7. A pregnant woman should not practice the Asana's from the 4th Month of her pregnancy.

8. Avoid performing Asana's back to back in quick succession, rest for at least 5-6 seconds between two Asana's.

9. After your Yoga session, do not eat or drink anything for at least 25 to 30 min.

10. If you have had a bone broken in the past and now its mended, still, don't submit that appendage to too much strain while performing an Asana.

11. Commit to routine practice of Yoga, make it a way of life.

Warm-up Exercises before you Begin

Like any other exercise, warming up before performing Yoga exercises (Asana's) is very important as it conditions your body to get used to the physical movements and stretching movements without bruising or hurting a muscle.

Look at the warm-up as an essential catalyst which enables your body to extract the full benefits of an Asana.

Warm-Up Exercise #1

Heel Raise:

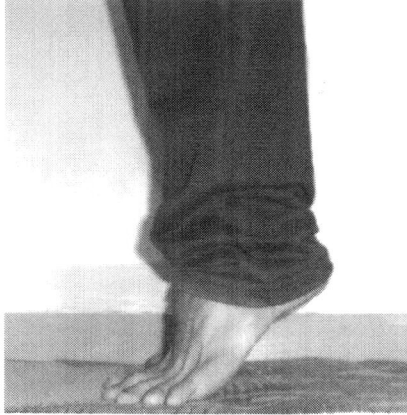

Stand straight/erect, without slouching.

Your feet should be close together.

Raise your body up on your toes (you can support yourself by holding on to a support).

Hold the position for 4-5 seconds and then slowly return to your original standing position.

Repeat it 7-8 times.

Advait

Warm-Up Exercise #2

Reverse Arch:

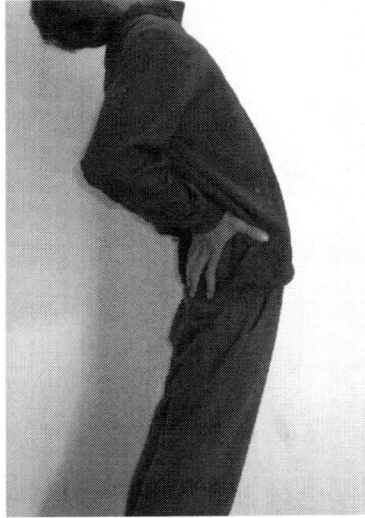

Stand straight/erect, without slouching.

Your feet should be around 1 foot apart.

Keep both your hands on your hips with your fingers pointing downwards.

Bend backwards at the waist, supporting your lower back with your hands.

(bend backwards as much as you can without hurting yourself)

Hold the position for 4-5 seconds and then slowly return to your original standing position.

Repeat it 5-6 times.

Warm-Up Exercise #3

Leg Raise:

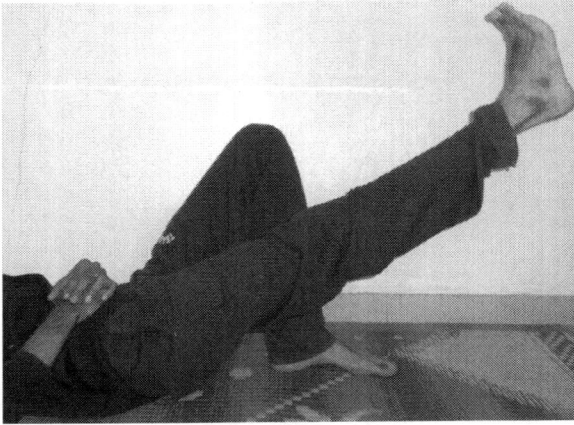

Lie on your back.

Keep one leg straight and the other bent at the knee.

Now slowly lift the straight leg up to a height of 10-12 inches from the ground and hold it there for 3-4 seconds.

Slowly take the raised leg down and repeat with the other leg.

This way, raise both the legs 7-8 times.

Warm-Up Exercise #4

Stretching Hamstring:

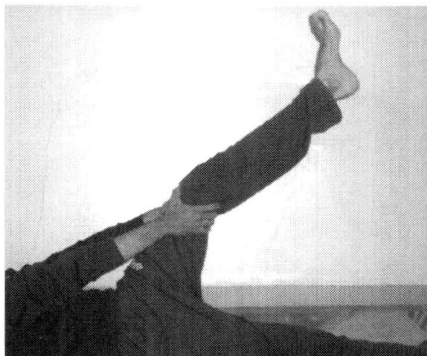

Lie on your back.

Keep one leg straight and the other bent at the knee.

Put your hands around the upper part of the bent leg. (refer image)

Slowly straighten the leg until you feel a stretch in the back of the upper leg and hold it for 3-4 seconds.

Slowly take the raised leg down and repeat with the other leg.

This way, raise both the legs 7-8 times.

Warm-Up Exercise #5

Single Knee Pull:

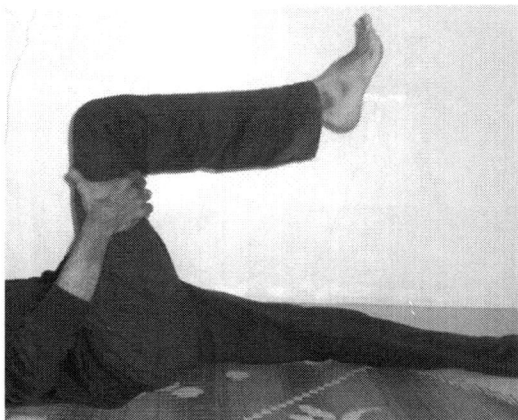

Lie on your back.

Keep one leg straight and the other bent at the knee.

Put your hands around the upper part of the bent leg. (refer image)

Now holding your thigh behind the knee, pull your knee up to your chest and hold for 3-4 seconds.

Slowly take the raised leg down and repeat with the other leg.

This way, raise both the legs 7-8 times.

Warm-Up Exercise #6

Double Knee Pull:

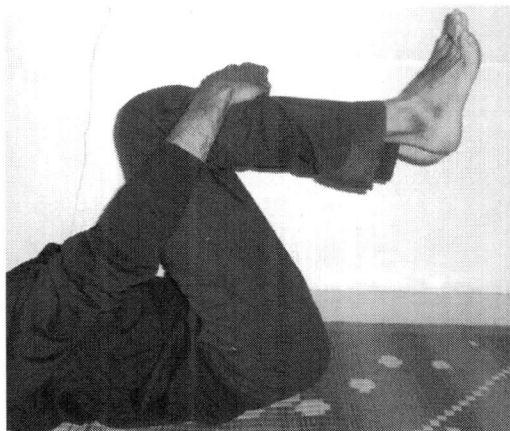

Lie on your back.

Keep both your legs bent at the knee.

Put your hands around the upper part of the bent legs. (refer image)

Now holding your thighs behind the knees, pull your knees up to your chest and hold for 3-4 seconds.

Slowly take the raised legs down.

Repeat for 7-8 times.

Advait

Warm-Up Exercise #7

Hip Roll:

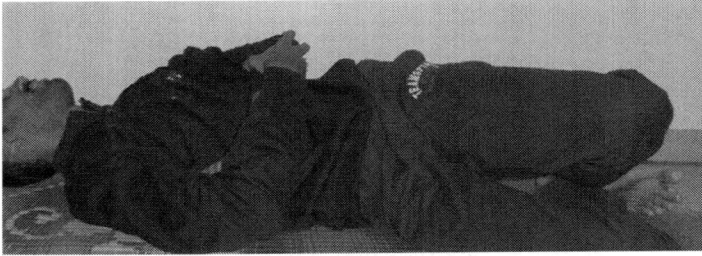

Lie on your back.

Keep both your legs bent at the knee.

Cross your arms over your chest.

Now, turn your head to the left while turning your knees to the right.

Invert and repeat.

10 Basic *Yoga Asana's* to get You started on the Path to Yoga

Yoga Asana #1

Swastikasan/Asana of Swastika

The Sanskrit word *Swastika* means pious. (do not confuse a swastika with the 'nazi symbol' which is an 'inverted' swastik)

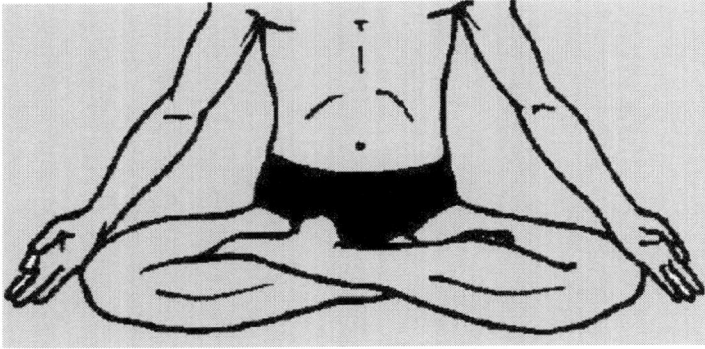

Method:

Sit comfortably on the mat.

Sit straight, with your spine erect. Do not slouch over.

Now fold your legs is such a way that the toes of your right foot are pressed between the thigh and calf muscle of the left leg and the toes of your left foot are pressed between the thigh and calf muscle of the right leg. (refer image)

Rest your hands on your knees, with your palms facing upwards.

Touch the tip of the index finger to the tip of the thumb on both your hands. (this hand gesture is called a *'Dnyanmudra'*)

Keep breathing slowly and comfortably while you perform this Asana.

Duration:

This Asana (position) should be held for 2-3 minutes.

Repeat at least 3 times for best results.

Uses:

-This Asana enhances mental strength

-It helps in calming down your mind.

-It strengthens your nervous system.

-On the physical front, This Asana helps in keeping Diabetes under control.

-It also strengthens the Pancreas.

Advait

Yoga Asana #2

Padmasan/ Asana of Lotus

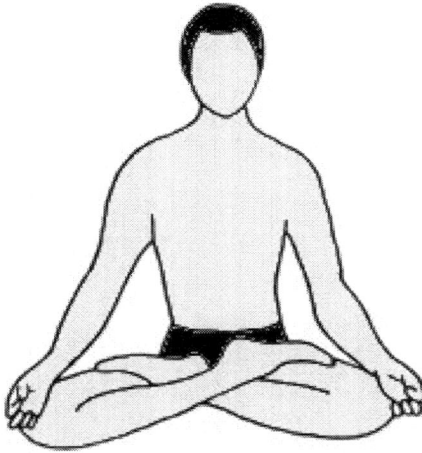

Method:

Sit comfortably on the mat with your legs stretched out front.

Now, fold your right leg and place the foot on your left thigh with the base of the right foot (palm of the foot) facing upwards. (refer the image)

Then, fold your left leg and place the foot on your right thigh with the base of the left foot (palm of the foot) facing upwards.

The heel of both your feet should be touching the base of the opposite thighs.

Rest your hands on your knees, with your palms facing upwards.

Touch the tip of the Index finger to the tip of the Thumb on both your hands.

Keep breathing slowly and comfortably while you perform this Asana.

(You will feel some pain when you are just starting out but with 4-5 days of regular practice, you should feel no discomfort.)

Duration:

When you perform this Asana for the first few days, do it only for 8-10 seconds at a stretch. But, with practice you'll fell more supple and flexible and then perform it for 1-2 minutes at a stretch.

Uses:

-It works miraculously well in treating Arthritis.

- It enhances your digestive capabilities.

Advait

- It cures any stomach aches you have and increase hunger.

-It strengthens your heart.

-It imparts flexibility to all the organs below the waistline.

-Regular practice of this Asana induces mental & spiritual calmness.

Yoga Asana #3

Taulasan/Asana of Scales

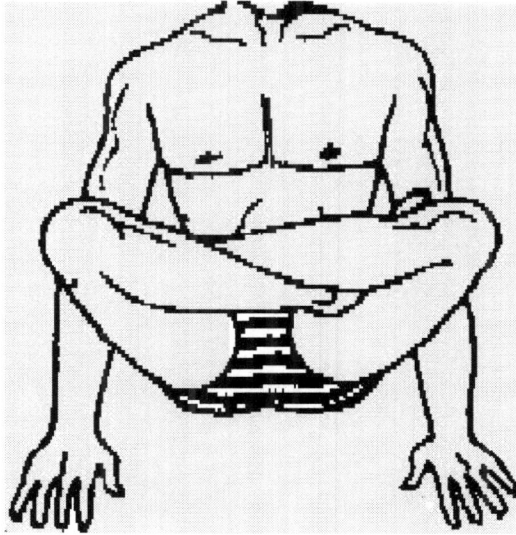

Method:

Sit comfortably on the mat with your legs stretched out front.

Now, fold your right leg and place the foot on your left thigh with the base of the right foot (palm of the foot) facing upwards. (refer the image)

Then, fold your left leg and place the foot on your right thigh with the base of the left foot (palm of the foot) facing upwards.

The heel of both your feet should be touching the base of the opposite thighs.

Keep both of your hands on the ground with your palms facing down.

Take a deep breath and don't exhale. (*Kumbhak*)

Now raise yourself up from the ground by putting all your weight on your hands. (refer image)

Hold this position for 3-4 seconds, then return to the normal position and exhale out slowly.

Duration:

This Asana takes 10-12 seconds to perform and you can repeat it 4-5 times.

Uses:

-This Asana strengthens your arms.

-It is very effective in curing back pain and shoulder pain.

-This is a very effective Asana for who those need to continuously type something sitting at their desk in their line of work. (writers, data -entry professionals etc.)

Yoga Asana #4

Parvatasan/Asana of Mountain

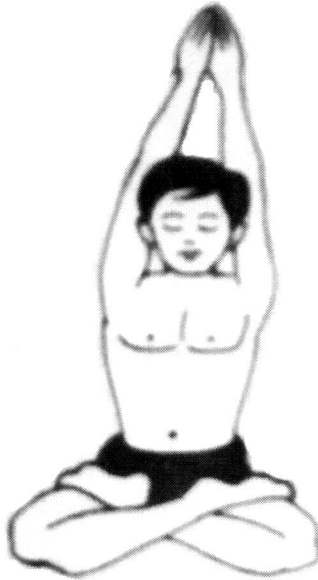

Method:

Sit comfortably on the mat with your legs stretched out front.

Now, fold your right leg and place the foot on your left thigh with the base of the right foot (palm of the foot) facing upwards. (refer the image)

Then, fold your left leg and place the foot on your right thigh with the base of the left foot (palm of the foot) facing upwards.

The heel of both your feet should be touching the base of the opposite thighs. (This is how you sit in *Padmasan*)

Now raise your hands up above your head and bring your palms together form a *Namaste* gesture (refer the image). [Namaste – Indian form of Salutation]

Extend your arms up, as much as you can without breaking the contact between your palms.

Take a deep breath, keep the air in for a few seconds and then exhale slowly. Bring your hands down and be in the original position.

All the while keep your body straight and aligned.

Duration:

This Asana takes 10-52 seconds to perform and you can repeat it 5-6 times.

Uses:

-This Asana strengthens the Muscles of your chest, abdomen and upper back.

-It is very helpful in strengthening the spinal chord.

-It's regular practice enhances one's digestive capabilities.

-It keeps your nervous system healthy.

-It is also found to be very helpful in healing stomach aches.

[End of Excerpt]

Want to read the entire book??

Buy it here:

http://www.amazon.com/dp/B010I97366

Printed in Great Britain
by Amazon